Help, Bette!

Answers to Health Questions from Hurting People

Bette Dowdell

HELP, BETTE!
Health Questions from
Hurting People

published by
Confident Faith Institute LLC
PO Box 11744
Glendale AZ 85318

http://BetteDowdell.com

First Print Edition

Printed in the U.S.A.

ISBN#: 978-0-9889953-3-8

Bette Dowdell is not a medical professional of any sort; she is a patient who researched her way out of a very deep health ditch when professionals failed.

Contents

Preface

Figuring out what's best for our health is a puzzlement.

I mean, it's not like we don't get plenty of information. We're awash in information—most of which is wrong.

The old saying goes, "After you hit a certain age, it's patch, patch, patch!" But it doesn't have to be that way. In fact, it shouldn't be that way.

Our bodies are intended to last. To serve us well until the end of our days. So why isn't that happening?

Two main reasons: We starve our bodies and we abuse our bodies.

Starving our bodies

"Starving? You say I'm starving? Oh, yeah, well just watch the scale get up and run away in terror when I show up!"

http://BetteDowdell.com

Well, most of us do worry more about losing weight than how gain a few pounds. But I'm not talking weight. I'm talking about making sure the body gets what it needs to thrive. I'm talking nutrition. All day, every day.

Not the nutrition of magazines, TV shows and doctors, but real nutrition. One-size-fits-all nutrition can't begin to meet our very individual needs.

Abusing our bodies

You already know drinking, smoking, staying up too late, taking illegal drugs (or any drugs, for that matter) doesn't do you any good. But at least you know what you're up against with that stuff.

Even worse are the secret toxins that jump up and down on our health—all while we don't even realize they're trouble with a capital T. Things like government-encouraged toxins such as fluoridated water, vaccines, bogus estrogen as far as the eye can see, fire-retardants, and on and on.

Not to mention the prescription medicines that do more harm than good.

As I answer questions, I'll be talking a lot about all of the above.

Where did these questions come from?

I offer a weekly health e-mail, *Too Pooped To Participate*. The free subscription includes a monthly teleseminar, often in the Q&A format. (The Resources chapter has a link you can use to subscribe.)

The questions in this book are just a few that subscribers have sent in. So, the questions come from real people, hurting people, perhaps even frightened people, wondering if it's even possible to get out of the ditch they're in.

I should probably tell you that my approach to health is different. Good health isn't about patching. It's about understanding how our bodies are supposed to work and what to do if they're going astray.

Even with just these few questions, chances are I'll contradict a lot of what you "know." In my struggle for health, I learned early on that sticking to conventional wisdom means defeat. Only persistent digging for truth allowed me to win my battle.

This book won't answer all your questions. Not even close. But it will introduce to a new way of thinking about your health.

http://BetteDowdell.com

I don't tell you what to do. Instead, I provide information you need to take control of your health—what symptoms mean, what can help, and what hurts.

Symptoms are your body's way of telling you what's wrong, and you're the only person in the universe that knows what your symptoms are.

Once you understand what your symptoms mean and match that up with how things are supposed to work, you're ready to start climbing out of the ditch.

This understanding-symptoms approach is the only way to get the custom-fit answer your body needs. And deserves.

Best of all, your body wants to heal. In fact, it fights like a tiger to heal, and once you start giving it the help it needs, your body turns into a healing machine.

It happened to me, and it can happen to you.

God is good,
Bette Dowdell
"Bette" has two syllables.
"Dowdell" rhymes with "cowbell"

Now, on with the questions.

http://BetteDowdell.com

Thyroid and Hair

"My blood test show I have low thyroid. I have had hair loss-I look like a cancer victim, with only a few hairs on my head. Before I started treatment a year ago I had enough hair for three people. Do you know how to get my hair back? I just decided to stop my synthroid to see if hair returns. Linda in Oklahoma."

Oh, I hear you, Linda. I used to actually cry when I looked in my bathroom mirror–and saw my scalp, shiny and bright under what hair remained–all the way to the back of my head.

The doctors' lack of answers–about my hair and lots of other problems–told me loud and clear that it was up to me if I expected anything good to happen.

That was the start of my years of research. And the beginning of getting my hair and my health back.

So, I'll start by telling you not to give up. Never.

Now let's talk.

Hair loss comes along with most endocrine problems. Where you lose hair varies by gland, but they all seem to head for the scalp.

The thyroid is part of the endocrine system, a little-known gang of glands that controls our health. And it's a gang that lives out the motto, "One for all, and all for one," all day, all night, all our lives.

When one of the gang goes down–in this case, your thyroid–all the others jump in to help. They can stagger along for a while, but if help doesn't arrive, they falter and fail.

So your thyroid gland may not be the only one in trouble.

But maybe it's not the thyroid at all. The problem may be an allergy to the Synthroid you took.

Synthroid doesn't treat low thyroid problems. To get a patent–and the big, big bucks–pharmaceutical companies stripped out one of the five parts of natural thyroid hormone, twisted it like a pretzel and pronounced it to be the answer.

Well, no. What with all that stripping and twisting, your body doesn't recognize Synthroid. Doesn't know what to do with it, in fact. And that goes for all T4 medicines.

So, although medicine swears Synthroid is the answer to everything, it doesn't work.

Worse, you can be allergic to it. Your hair loss may be an allergic reaction. Stopping for a while is a good idea.

Or it may be you have a nutrition problem. And, yes, thyroid tests are unreliable enough to say you have a problem when you don't.

For instance, if you live on the low-fat diet so beloved by poobahs and the media, you're killing your thyroid–and all the other members of the endocrine gang.

Your body makes its endocrine hormones from saturated fat. Your brain is mostly sat fat, too. A low-fat diet invites disaster.

As you can see, problems and answers aren't black-and-white simple. Getting the endocrine system back on the straight and narrow takes a lot of information–how things are supposed to work, what our symptoms mean, etc.

Determining if Synthroid caused your hair loss is a good start. Getting your nutrition lined up for health will pay off, no matter what.

http://BetteDowdell.com

Kidney Disease

"Hi Bette. I'm in stage 4 kidney disease from bilateral polycystic kidneys. Now, I'm not on dialysis and don't want to be. I suffer from occasional gout attacks (big toe, ankle, elbow from high uric acid levels), painful boils & what's so strange is they come either all over on the right side or on the left side. in the groin, under arm, breast, buttock, stomach even. What's that about and what can I do to prevent them? Very painful. I'm currently taking Losartan 100mg for high blood, Bumetenide for a diuretic, Calcitriol for vitamin d, and Nephrocaps as a vitamin. I suffer from palpitations occasionally, all-over joint pain, headaches, rashes on my neck, lethargy, tiredness (am anemic also), fatigue and weakness feeling. I'm a mess sometimes. I was put on a 70gr /day protein diet. I try to stick to it. I also have a goiter on my thyroid and am hypo on no meds at this time for it. I think my immune system is suffering also cause I can sometimes feel a lump right under my chin and was told it was a lymph gland? my creatinine level is at 3.9, gfr is 15, platelet count is over 500, it's just awful. Please help. I don't want to start dialysis. I'm on the national organ transplant register for just 1-1/2 yrs

so far. I was told because I'm O+, I have a 4-5 yr wait. Thanks for your time - Robin"

As you all can see, our girl, Robin, is in a world of hurt. Things look pretty grim.

But, thanks to our fabulous bodies, there's always hope—if you know what to do to help your body make a break for health.

So let's step through the information we have and look for clues.

- Polycystic kidneys means her kidneys are dealing with lots of cysts. Cysts point to an iodine deficiency.

- Gout often shows up when high fructose corn syrup keeps slip-sliding down the gullet.

- Boils are a big-time way your body screams for nutrition.

- Heart palpitations usually mean at least some of your body's epithelial cells are in trouble, another nutritional problem.

- Goiter points to an underperforming thyroid; it means the body needs more nutrition, including iodine.

- Low thyroid function brings along anemia as a symptom.

http://BetteDowdell.com

- When any part of the endocrine system goes down, the rest of the gang jumps in to help. It usually ends up badly–and the immune system, which is a member of the endocrine gang, gets whacked.

Meanwhile, what's the doc doing?
- The blood pressure medicine, Losartan, protects the kidneys in diabetic patients.

- The powerful diuretic, Bumetanide, is suggested for cases of heart failure, with a note to tell the doctor if you have liver or kidney disease.

- Calcitriol is an inferior form of vitamin D.

- The multi, Nephrocaps, offers tiny little dabs of a few vitamins–some in inferior forms. Besides offering virtually no nutrition, Nephrocaps contain soy, titanium dioxide and food colorings–none of which should pass anybody's lips.

So what should Robin do?
First and foremost, Robin should take responsibility for her own health. She's the one with the most "skin in the game," as the saying goes, so she's the one who needs to act.

Fluoride is a well known cause of kidney disease, and Robin lives in Philadelphia, which started fluoridating the water in 1954.

http://BetteDowdell.com

One writer, with advanced kidney disease similar to Robin's, reports she cut her GFR (blood test reading) level by half in four months just by avoiding fluoride. Upon recovering her health, she took to crusading against the stuff. Good for her!

So Robin should not drink fluoridated water, cook with it, bathe in it, shower in it, swim in it or let it into her body any other way.

High fructose corn syrup not only causes gout, but also damages the kidneys. Robin should eliminate high fructose corn syrup from her diet. It's everywhere, so avoiding it takes attention, but restoring health merits whatever effort it takes.

In fact, until the kidneys are once again singing and dancing, she should avoid all fructose, including that in fruit, fruit juices, agave syrup, etc.

Vitamins and minerals are serious business. The media, the talking heads, etc. pooh-pooh nutritional supplements, but good supplements (unlike Nephrocaps) lead to good health. However, there's a lot to learn about them to do it right, so I write about that.

These actions will address most, if not all, of Robin's problems. Life doesn't come with guarantees, but she should see a remarkable difference.

http://BetteDowdell.com

How to proceed

Robin can act on her own by avoiding both fluoride and high fructose corn syrup.

She can also act on her own in starting a solid vitamin/mineral program that takes her kidney disease into consideration.

Beyond what Robin can do on her own, it's good for patients to inform the doctor about what they're doing. However, that's not always possible, and Robin will have to play it by ear. What she doesn't need is a hostile doc.

There's a lot more to say about the care and healing of the kidneys, and I say it in my *Moving to Health* program.

Bottom line: Take responsibility for your own health, live long and prosper.

http://BetteDowdell.com

Statins and Diabetes

"Hi Bette: I have a slight heart problem and the same for diabetes. I am on some statins for the heart and it is my wish to get completely off of them before too much more time passes. Do you have a recommendation about going off the statins? I control the diabetes so far with some supplements. Thanks ever so much. Charles"

Hi, Charles,

If you study history, you'll remember that the Father of Our Country, George Washington, was killed by standard medical practice.

The preferred treatment of the day—for almost everything—was "bleeding," drawing off significant amounts of blood because they believed toxins lived in the blood, and getting rid of blood got rid of toxins.

Well, now, there's an oops. They bumped off a lot of folks, including George Washington, with this misguided treatment.

Today's hot-shot medical treatment, statin drugs, is as misguided as bleeding. And also kills a lot of patients. A recent study labeled statins as the greatest medical fraud of all time.

So I understand your wanting to get off statins. They're hard on the body. They whack your endocrine system, do a job on your brain, cause aches and pains that pretty much ruin your quality of life, and on, and on.

Statins skyrocket your risk of diseases of all sorts.

For instance, statins cause diabetes. And heart attacks. And congestive heart failure. And various autoimmune diseases. Cancer. And I could go on.

And all that risk is for nothing. Statins aim at the wrong target. Cholesterol doesn't cause heart problems. I repeat, cholesterol does NOT cause heart problems.

In fact, people with "high" cholesterol (200 to 308–which is as high as they tested) lived longer, healthier lives.

On the other hand, low cholesterol is a killer. A total cholesterol level of less than 180 flirts shamelessly with disease. Below 150, and you're sending engraved invitations to cancer and other bad actors. And when your cholesterol slides under 120, you're going down.

So, what causes heart disease? Inflammation. In fact, inflammation causes most diseases.

And while medicine has nothing to offer to treat inflammation, it can be handled nicely with vitamins and minerals.

Nutrition puts muscle in your fight with diabetes, too. In fact, studies are showing up that prove good nutrition, including your diet, can actually reverse diabetes.

For diet, avoid grains and carbs, get plenty of Omega 3 saturated fat and a good amount of protein.

For vitamins and minerals, etc., check out the Resources chapter.

Sorry to hear you're having to deal with this stuff. You must feel like a truck hit you.

http://BetteDowdell.com

Liver Problems

"I have never really done low fat, but recently, my doctor wanted me to take Zocor because she thought my levels were too high because of prediabetes, I took it for 2 days and my legs hurt so much I stopped. My glucose levels shot up to the 300's while I was on this. Yesterday I had blood levels taken and my cholesterol levels are up and my A1C is higher!! Would healing my liver help glucose and cholesterol levels? Chromium is not good for the liver. I don't know which one to concentrate on. Liver or glucose or cholesterol. Corinne from Colorado"

Holy Moley, Corinne! You're in a mess, which you did nothing to deserve.

Let's talk about this.

First off, statin drugs–Zocor and all the rest–do absolutely nothing for the female of the species. Zip, zero, nada.

In fact, for females, statin drugs are only about side effects. Bad side effects. Men get a teensy-tinesy, hard-to-notice benefit from statins, but women get only problems. Nobody should take statin drugs, but especially women.

As you found out the hard way.

As I said in the last chapter, statin drugs cause diabetes. So your doctor decided you were prediabetic and put you on statins? Was she afraid you wouldn't become diabetic quickly enough? Yikes!

Forget all the tests and test results until your body has a chance to recover from the statin insult.

And ignore cholesterol, now and ever after.

Healing your liver, though, is a swell idea. Fatty liver disease, the innocent-sounding name for non-alcoholic cirrhosis, is epidemic nowadays.

Cirrhosis destroys the liver. No liver function means death, which is never good news.

But with proper nutrition (medicine has nothing to offer), even an 80% destroyed liver can be restored to health.

So I vote for the liver. Restoring the liver is one of the many things covered in my *Moving to Health* program.

http://BetteDowdell.com

Healing the liver isn't hard, but given our complicated bodies where everything affects everything else, there are a lot of moving parts to know about.

http://BetteDowdell.com

Cholesterol and Statin Drugs

"Hi I am female. Age 58. Menopause since 54. On synthroid 17 years. Dose 0.088mg. Fighting high cholesterol since menopause. Did have LDL down to 3.82 but 6 months later it is again up to 4.90 (Canadian numbers) Doctor wants me to go on Lipitor or Crestor. I am fighting him on this. I am in great shape, low blood pressure, non smoker, non drinker, diet is very very good, and I exercise every day. Please advise me with help to lower and keep down LDL and how to tell the doctor that I am not going on Lipitor!!!!!!! Thank you so much!! Debbie from Newfoundland, Canada"

You're right, and the doc's wrong in this one.

So you have to stand up big and tall, look the doc right in the eye and say, "NO!"

This is hard to do, especially when we've been raised as good little girls who don't talk back to those in authority. All the certificates on the wall and the stethoscope around the doctor's neck make it even harder. But it has to be done.

Best case, you'll start a new kind of relationship with the doctor, a type of partnership.

Worse case–and this is more likely, unfortunately–the doctor fires you as a patient.

This kind of sounds like a disaster, but think it through. Do you want to stay with a doctor who won't listen to you? Who insists on prescribing drugs that harm you?

Especially since you do so very well on your own. And even more, since cholesterol is never the problem.

Besides, at age 58, isn't it about time the doc treated you as an adult?

Full-Body Itching

"My mother is 94...has had an all over body itch for years...no one knows the answer...just had her liver duct cleaned out...did not help.....no noticeable allergies..nothing we have tried, lotions etc. make it better. Gail from Sidney, Australia"

There's not a lot of information to work with in this question. Which is a little daunting since even the hands-on people don't have a clue about what's going on.

But while I can't read tea leaves, I can make some educated guesses and suggestions—none of which will do harm in any case.

The itch almost surely comes from a systemic problem. Something got started and followed the path of least resistance to wiggle and squirm its way to where it doesn't belong.

The result is itching, which really takes a lot of joy out of life.

http://BetteDowdell.com

I'll suggest two things to try. One for the inside, and one for the outside.

For the inside, I suggest *Carlson's Lemon-Flavored Cod Liver Oil*. It contains high quality Omega 3 fats; itching is often a sign of a an Omega 3 fat deficiency.

Additionally, Vitamin D3 and natural Vitamin A come along for the ride, and they'll give your mother a boost. Plus, itching can come from a Vitamin A deficiency.

Some people worry about taking natural Vitamin A, but Vitamin D balances those worries away.

And this cod liver oil tastes good. Mothers even report that little babies slurp it up with delight.

As with everything, start slowly. Maybe a half-teaspoon once a day for a week. Then a full teaspoon once a day. Then a full teaspoon twice a day.

Keep checking in with her about how it makes her feel. Our bodies tell us when enough is enough, so ask your mother to share that information with you.

For the outside, try *Life-Flo's MSMPlus*, a pump-bottle lotion. It's sold to ease joint pain, but it's also great for the skin. Some people use it as a daily moisturizer.

http://BetteDowdell.com

You can get both the cod liver oil and the MSM lotion online.

I pray that my suggestions hit the nail on the head, as the saying goes, so your mom gets relief.

At 94, she deserves a break. And you do, too.

http://BetteDowdell.com

Dry Eye

"I was diagnosed with a flareup of dry eyes which is very uncomfortable. Could there be a connection to the thyroid? I am very tired most of the time and have other symptoms pointing to an under active thyroid. My TSH test is fine, and my doctor tells me I do not need the Armour. But my eye problem persists. I am 79 years old. The doctor prescribed Restasis drops in the eyes to calm down the inflammation and to encourage tear production. I am hesitating to use them. Gisela from California"

You're a wise woman, Gisela.

The TSH test may be the least reliable test in the history of medicine. If not the worst, it's at least a contender.

Part of the problem comes from the wide "normal" range. You want to be in the low end of the "reference range" that defines normal, but even that's not a guarantee of reliability.

The symptoms always tell the story. Symptoms are your body's way of letting you know what's going on.

http://BetteDowdell.com

Helping your body with the vitamins, minerals, etc. it needs should moderate the symptoms. Might even overcome them. Since your doctor chooses not to help, that looks like the path to take.

Let me tell you a story about my experience with dry eye.

My left eye had an unfortunate encounter with a dead palm tree branch, which tore the cornea. You want to talk about pain! Whoa, baby! A torn cornea gets your full attention.

And it wouldn't heal because of my dry eye. During the night, whenever I went into REM (rapid eye movement) sleep, my cornea would get torn again. Night after night.

It wasn't the most fun I ever had. Sound asleep, minding my own business, and all of a sudden, it felt like somebody was stabbing me in the eye.

The doctor treating my cornea was the head of ophthalmology at the University of Arizona medical school and a cornea specialist. He labeled my problem as Cogan's Dystrophy and said it would never go away.

He videotaped my eye to create a teaching tool. Apparently, real live cases of Cogan's are rare, and he wanted students to see what it looked like "in action."

The mess went on for months—until a regular appointment with my dentist. He took one look at my swollen, leaking eye and said I needed evening primrose oil. I borrowed one of his alternative health books to read about it.

It only took about a week to get results. Years later, because I live in a dry climate, I still take evening primrose oil.

On my next visit to the ophthalmologist, I announced (with great fanfare, I must say) that I was healed.

He disagreed and tried to find the tear in the cornea, but couldn't. Even when looking through the king of all magnifying glasses.

He asked what I had been doing, but when I mentioned the evening primrose oil, he said oil had nothing to do with anything, and I was just lucky. Really nice guy, but way too opinionated.

All that said, you might want to try evening primrose oil. It has a long, strong history of reversing dry eye problems.

I take Solgar's Evening Primrose Oil, 1300mg once or twice a day.

Prostate Cancer

"Dear Bette, My brother has been diagnosed with prostate cancer which has spread to the bone. They are not doing any surgery but he is getting a shot of a drug that contains estrogen. I don't understand how this is supposed to slow the cancer growth. I have a problem with this making sense as I wonder if he has low testosterone. The only diet recommendation is to not eat sugar foods. Thank you. Joan from Wisconsin"

Oh, Joan, I am so sorry.

Prescribing estrogen for prostate cancer is another failed medical experiment. The news is spreading that estrogen is exactly the wrong thing to give to prostate cancer patients, but it'll take years for it to get to the local doctor.

Even though it makes no sense, the theory is prostate cancer is caused by too much testosterone, and the estrogen treatment gets rid of devil testosterone.

But I ask you: If too much testosterone were the problem, why aren't teen-age boys dropping like flies?

Because of the treatment he received, your brother is in trouble. Real trouble.

After the estrogen treatment, once the cancer gets in the bones, heroic measures are called for.

He needs massive doses of vitamins, minerals, etc. Given the trouble he's in, his body will slurp up what you give him with joy. Don't worry about overdoses—at least for a while.

For example, Carlson's lemon-flavored cod liver oil through the day. A B100 Complex at least three times a day. TwinLabs Daily One multi without iron at least three times a day. Lots of free-form glutamine—at least 40 grams a day. And so on.

It would be wonderful if you can find a doctor who gives Vitamin C intravenously. That way your brother would get the necessary, massive doses that aren't possible with oral supplements. Mainline doctors don't do this; you'll have to go alternative—which is what you want here.

Get all the estrogen out of his life: Grocery store meat and milk, canned foods, soy, flax, fragrances, etc. And, of course, the estrogen-laced meds the doctor's giving him have to go.

Try to find a doctor who will give your brother testosterone. Not all doctors will take a patient with prostate cancer that's metastasized to the bone, so this may take a real hunt.

This is literally a fight for your brother's life, so don't hold back. Give it everything you have. And don't wait to act.

Nothing I suggested will interfere with chemotherapy, but will, in fact, enhance it.

As you know, I'm not a doctor or medical professional of any sort. What I offer is my 30+ years of research–and my concern.

I lost a wonderful brother because of the misguided estrogen treatment.

http://BetteDowdell.com

IBS - Irritable Bowel Syndrome

"Hi Bette, thanks for your show and sharing your knowledge. I subscribe to your newsletter and love your work. Are you able to tell me what I can do for histamine intolerance? I've had IBS for 25+ years and I think this recent diagnoses hits the mark. I have been tested and results came back that I have a DAO [diamine oxidase] *deficiency. I am also aware of a number of food sensitivities but can't seem to tolerate probiotics to repair my gut, this is due to the fermentation process. I am on a strict diet. There is a genetic link as my father and sister suffer to some degree also. I believe in epigenics and understand that it is possible to turn off DNA expressions and control symptoms. Please offer your valued opinion as I respect your level of experience. Matthew from Melbourne, Australia"*

Thanks for your kind words, Matthew. I hope you don't change your opinion when I say it appears you're working with a bogus diagnosis.

A diagnosis that was developed, mainly by dietitians, based on mistaking correlations with causes. These are the same folks

http://BetteDowdell.com

who promote the low-fat diet that speeds us on our way to disease.

IBS (irritable bowel syndrome) develops when the epithelial lining of the small intestine gets ruptured and allows half-digested foods out of the intestine into body parts that can't handle it. The body reacts to the insult, sometimes pretty forcefully, as you know.

And how does the epithelial lining get breached? Low stomach acid (which I write about elsewhere in this book), a whacked endocrine system and fluoride are the main culprits.

Fluoride is industrial waste, a poison. It makes stomach acid and endocrine problems worse, much worse.

But don't expect the poobahs to come out against fluoride. Fluoride creates patients. Medicine won't blow the whistle on this gravy train.

So, they come up with a diagnosis like DAO deficiency, for which they have no treatment. Which leaves you to suffer on and on.

For instance, you've been dealing with IBS, and all its food sensitivities, for more than 25 years. There is a cure, and I lay it all out in my *Moving to Health* program. The fix isn't difficult, but it also isn't obvious or easy–there are a lot of

http://BetteDowdell.com

moving parts–and it takes some effort. But it ends the IBS mess by repairing the intestinal lining. Talk about happy endings!

Finally, a damaged small intestine can't utilize probiotics while it's fighting for its life. Fermentation isn't the problem. Your body's yelling "Out! Out!" because it's in too much of a mess to deal with outsiders.

Now let's discuss the mistaken message about histamine that gets bandied about with the DAO diagnosis.

Histamine is your friend. I may be the only person you'll hear say that, but it's a fact.

First, some background.

Amino acids enable our bodies to be all they can be. One such amino acid is histidine. All aminos are important, with histidine more so than some others.

One histidine action is creating histamine when the body's under attack from allergens. Histamine protects our body parts from damage.

But some sneezing and honking may go on, so people see a histamine reaction as a bad thing. And here come antihistamines down the gullet.

http://BetteDowdell.com

Now there's an oops! Histamine gives everything it has to protect us, while antihistamines shout, "Oh, no you don't!"

While antihistamines give us temporary relief, they whack our bodies something fierce—which we don't realize. What we do notice, often without making a connection, is antihistamines cause us to gain weight.

By now you may be asking "If histamine, histidine, amino acids and all the rest are so important, why don't we hear about them? "

Medical schools don't teach a word about amino acids—not what they are or what they do. Doctors know drugs, but not nutrition. So they know how to push the body around, but not how to help it heal.

Pharmaceutical companies can't match amino acids, and they can't patent them, either. So, they're against them.

Magazines, TV, etc. don't cover anything that pharmaceutical companies don't like. And doctors have to go along or risk their medical license.

But there is a cure for you. Not just a patch, but a cure.

Kids and Hashimoto's

"Hello Bette, All three of my children ages 6, 10, & 12, have been diagnosed with Hashimotos, and have highly elevated antibody levels. I was also diagnosed very young at age 13, now 38 years old. What can we do to help them prevent the progression of the disease? A gluten free diet has been advised, and they have begun taking Wobenzym N systemic enzymes. Please help, as I am overwhelmed and desperately want to help them and not have to have them go through the lifetime of suffering that I have from thyroid disease. Why are so many children being diagnosed now? What else can we do as parents? Thank you so very much.   Nicole from Delaware"

I'm so sorry you have to deal with all of this, Nicole. Fighting your own battle is tough enough, but seeing your kids in trouble is worse. Especially when answers are so hard to come by.

That said, the diagnosis gives me more questions than answers. So let me run through some random thoughts for you to consider.

http://BetteDowdell.com

1. What looks like Hashimoto's may actually be nutritional deficiencies. Some people tell me that following my vitamin/mineral program "cured" their Hashimoto's.

   The more likely reality is nutritional deficiencies were misdiagnosed as Hashimoto's, and removing the deficiencies was the answer.

2. Following the low-fat diet touted by dietitians leaves the thyroid–the entire endocrine system for that matter–gasping for air and screaming for help.

   And not just any fat will do. Avoid vegetable oils, partially hydrogenated or not. (Olive oil's okay as long as you don't cook with it.)

   What we need is saturated fat. Our bodies make all their endocrine hormones–thyroid, insulin, cortisol, estrogen, etc.–from saturated fat. Our brains are mostly saturated fat.

   I know, I know, we all hear that saturated fat is the worst enemy of all time, but good old sat fat is really a dandy, tried-and-true friend.

   Again, not just any sat fat. The meat and milk they sell in grocery stores is loaded with antibiotics and hormones. Plus the fat's not even close to what it should be.

http://BetteDowdell.com

So stick with meat and milk from grass-fed cows, free-range chickens, etc. Add some organic coconut oil for a nice pick-me-up.

3. Fluoride stomps on the thyroid and causes antibodies. It also makes kids passive and reduces their IQs. A pea-size glob of fluoridated toothpaste can kill a small child.

   Avoid all fluoride any way you can.

4. Wobenzym N enzymes are great, but in this case, they're more a matter of "doing something" than addressing the problem.

5. Your liver has to be in good shape for your thyroid to work. Your thyroid can pour out all the thyroid hormone you need, but a punk liver will keep your body from using it.

So there are five major things to consider in your search for health.

Prostate Questions

"Hi Bette, I am a 77 yr old male. Last PSA test was elevated-again. Number was about 7.02. Also exam showed enlarged prostrate. Many conflicting reports out there. Any help? Richardo from Wisconsin"

Let's talk about this, Richardo.

First off, you'll want to know that the doctor who developed the PSA test now wishes he hadn't because it's being misused.

And there's so much kick-back from unreliable outcomes, inappropriate treatment and the like, labs now offer age-related results. Since PSA levels can rise as birthdays go by, this makes sense.

One lab gave the following levels:
- Younger than 50: PSA should be less than 2.5.
- 50 to 59: PSA should be less than 3.5.
- 60 to 69: PSA should be less than 4.5
- Older than 70: PSA should be less than 6.5

Those levels may or may not have anything to do with anything. But, even so, if the acceptable PSA level increases by 1 each decade, then you're right about where you should be, less than 7.5. But nobody really knows.

Jeffrey Dach, MD, wrote, "PSA screening for prostate cancer is, in fact, a 20-year failed medical experiment which provides little or no benefit in saving lives."

In terms of the enlarged prostate, age can increase prostate size, especially without good nutrition. The really inconvenient thing about an enlarged prostate is the time spent in the bathroom. Inconvenient, but not necessarily dangerous.

If bathroom visits include urgency and pain, it may be interstitial cystitis. Again, not dangerous, but certainly not a walk in the park. The fix is nutritional, not medical.

You're wise to keep track of where your body's going, but don't be afraid of normal results, even if they're presented as an invitation to doom.

And don't accept them as inevitable and unchangeable, either.

For every health problem known to mankind, my first suggestion is (and always will be) to build a solid vitamin/mineral program for yourself. Not a little bit of this and a little bit of that, but a solid program that specifically fulfills your body's needs.

Amino acids and other supplements work their specific wonders, too, but just getting vitamins and minerals right puts you ahead of the pack.

Anybody who bases their vitamin/mineral intake on what they read in magazines, hear on TV, etc. is going down. That's why I write my books and programs.

There's an herb that deals with enlarged prostates, Stinging Nettle root, usually just called Nettle Root. You can get Nettle Leaf supplements, too, but they don't help the prostate.

Finally, fluoride—in the water, in Coca Cola, in Nestle's bottled water, in toothpaste, in mouthwash, wherever—sets the stage for disease, including prostate cancer and interstitial cystitis. Avoid fluoride.

So there you have it: Give your body the nutrition it needs and avoid both estrogen and fluoride. It's easier to say than do, but not complicated.

http://BetteDowdell.com

Thyroid or Adrenal?

"I have had hypothyroidism for about 10 years, tests TSH FT3 and FT4 RT3, clearly show this. Regardless of trying synthroid, cytomel nature-throid, and all combinations I continue to suffer from fatigue and low body temp. I am starting to think that my condition may be more related to adrenal fatigue than thyroid. What do you think, and if you agree what can be done to treat this. Thank You!! PS I follow your advice in the program very closely Frank from Florida"

Well, Frank, the good news is that they even tested you. Thyroid is considered a "female" disease, so men rarely get tested. Even though it's not all that uncommon in men. So congratulations.

Of course, thyroid tests rank right up there among the really unreliable tests. It's symptoms that tell the story, and your symptoms say there's trouble.

Synthroid, even with Cytomel, lacks oomph. Cytomel helps, but not enough to really get the whole job done.

http://BetteDowdell.com

Naturethroid, a natural, bio-identical thyroid medication, is the real deal. However, relying on the unreliable tests, doctors rarely prescribe as much as you need. That may be at least a part of your problem.

Your suspicion of adrenal problems is right on the money. The thyroid and adrenals are partners in mischief, so both need to be checked–and treated.

In fact, the PDR (Physician's Desk Reference), the so-called bible of medical practice, says no thyroid meds should ever be prescribed until the adrenals are checked. But it happens all the time.

Of course, nowadays they check the adrenals via a blood test–signifying nothing.

Some years ago, two different doctors checked my adrenals–one with a blood test, the other with a saliva test–within a week of each other. The blood test said I was fine; the saliva test said I was in adrenal failure–as did my symptoms.

Doctors risk their medical license by ordering saliva tests (a rule set by insurance companies, as allowed by Congress), but you can get one at http://CanaryClub.org, a very reliable organization.

I took various meds and "supports" for the adrenals, without getting results. What did the job was a strong nutritional program, starting with vitamins and minerals.

Medicine pooh-poohs vitamins and minerals, but ignore those folks. Vitamins and minerals have the power and the glory we all need.

Hepatitis

"Hi, I am on Day 8 of a 30-day juice fast. I am 52 years old and have hepatitis C. I don't take any prescription medications. I feel fine with the fast so far. I have more energy, mind is clearer, and I'm sleeping better. Should I be taking supplements of any kind during this fast. Donna in Oklahoma"

Well, let's talk about a juice fast. Now, with hepatitis C, you already have trouble with your liver. Okay, you know that.

Your liver is hurting, it can't get rid of toxins as well as it should, and there are a lot of ramifications with hepatitis C.

The liver is usually fixable. I talk about how in the *Moving To Health* program. It's more than I can cover in a small book like this, but it's there if you're interested.

But meanwhile, I hope you're not drinking lots of fruit juices because fruit juices have fructose in them. And while natural fructose is not as bad as something like high-fructose corn syrup, it does demand a lot of the liver because the liver really doesn't know how to handle fructose.

Did you know that when sucrose (sugar) goes into your body, and fructose goes into your body, they are handled separately? Entirely separately.

Sugar will never be a health food, but at least every cell of the body knows how to react to sugar. Fructose, on the other hand, is a mystery to our cells—and not handled well.

So, if you get a lot of fructose – I talked to one guy who went on a juice fast with a lot of fructose. He did love fruit. You can't blame him; fruit tastes great. But he ended up with gout, a sure sign of too much fructose. So, I hope you're not getting heavily involved in fruit juices.

And if you are using reconstituted juices from concentrate, you need to know that chances are it was reconstituted with fluoridated water, which is, again, hard on the liver.

Some juices that are supposed to be good for the liver are beet juice, sometimes called beet root juice, and carrot juice.

Some people stay away from carrot because they say it has a high glycemic index, and it's too much sugar all at once. But they're finding out that the glycemic index needs some fine tuning, and carrot isn't so bad. Your body will be happy to offer its opinion.

So, should you be taking supplements? Oh, indeed. You should be taking a ton of supplements because if you want your body to heal, you have to give it what it needs. And it's not just, as I frequently say, the odd vitamin. You have to set up a whole program of quality supplements to give your body the nutrition it needs.

Acid Reflux

"What is the best medicine to take to prevent acid reflux? Give as much info as the time permits. Thanks, Bette. Frank in New York"

There's no good medicine for acid reflux. The medicines they have make things worse for lots of folks, and a lot of the meds are addictive.

Medicine says acid reflux means there's too much stomach acid, but the reality is that most people don't have enough.

The tricky thing is that high stomach acid and low stomach acid have the same symptoms–heartburn, bloating, burping, etc. And most cases of GERD as they call it–Gastro Esophageal Reflux–come from low stomach acid, also called hypochlorhydria.

Low stomach acid, not high, is usually the villain.

But all the ads about stomach acid teach us that high stomach acid is the only possible diagnosis. Ad after ad after ad says take this pill and your stomach acid goes away.

But for most of us, heartburn meds make things worse. We think they're helping but we have to take more and more to keep up, which is kind of the big clue.

And meanwhile, as our stomach acid levels drop lower and lower, we're destroying our innards. And our health.

Problems caused by low stomach acid

First off, you whack the endocrine system. The conditions that are caused or made worse by low stomach acid are (in no particular order here):

- Hashimoto's, an autoimmune version of thyroid problems.

- Other autoimmune diseases like rheumatoid arthritis, multiple sclerosis, lupus–all of them pretty much–are related to or made worse by low stomach acid.

- Vitiligo which is the white patches on the skin. That's what Michael Jackson had, and you'll read there's no treatment. But low stomach acid is a big-time cause of vitiligo. So that's something that you have to check.

- Another is high adrenal cortisol levels, causing all sorts of misery. If you have high cortisol levels and low stomach acid, eventually the adrenals just kind of give up and then you crash.

But it's not just the endocrine system that goes down in flames!

- Gall bladder problems are often caused by low stomach acid.

- Celiac disease which often accompanies endocrine problems, very, very often comes from low stomach acid.

- Colitis, an inflammation of the colon. Eighty percent of people suffering from colitis have low stomach acid.

- Ulcers, because when your stomach acid is low, bacteria like H pylori, which causes ulcers, can take over. That's another thing to check, although nobody does.

- Food sensitivities. Our stomach bloats. We get diarrhea. We throw up. We get rashes. We make unexpected mad dashes for the bathroom .

- And low stomach acid can make our blood acidic, which is a very bad thing.

- Low stomach acid causes rapid aging, chronic fatigue, B12 and mineral deficiencies, and anemia.

http://BetteDowdell.com

- Asthma. Maybe you had asthma as a kid and then grew out of it. Then as you got older, it came back. Well, a lot of little kids have trouble generating enough stomach acid, and so they get asthma. As they grow and mature, they grow out of it because they develop the stomach acid that they need. But then as they age, stomach acid levels drop and the asthma comes back.

- Okay, another is Reynaud's Phenomenon. I used to have that years ago as part of my endocrine journey. What happens is your extremities, your hands and your feet lose circulation if they get cold, and they look like a cadaver, to tell the truth, and they're numb. When the blood comes back in them, it hurts like you cannot believe.

- Rosacea.

- Candida.

And I could go on and on and on

Who gets hypochlorhydria?

- People over 35. Some books say over 45 but most say over 35.

- People who took antibiotics. It creates an overgrowth of bad bacteria, and after a while, there goes the acid.

- People who take heartburn medicine, whether prescription or over-the-counter.

- People who had gastric bypass surgery.

- Those on a poor diet of processed foods, high fructose corn syrup, sugar, white bread, etc.

Symptoms of low stomach acid
- Splitting and cracking fingernails can point to a stomach acid problem

- If your food looks pretty much the same coming out as it did going in, it can mean low stomach acid.

- You can get some dilated capillaries in your cheeks. Maybe just a few. They look like little worms, wiggly but not very big.

- Another symptom is bursitis.

- If you have an itchy rectum, think low stomach acid.

- If you have pain at the base of your thumbs, where your thumb joins side of your arm, that's probably low stomach acid.

http://BetteDowdell.com

What not to do:

Without enough stomach acid, you're unable to digest protein. If you can't digest protein, life gets hard and health chaos ensues.

It's from digested protein that our bodies create amino acids, which do about a gazillion wonderful things for our health.

And our bodies create enzymes–customized to our momentary needs–from amino acids, so no aminos means an enzyme shortage.

Taking enzymes is not the answer because they're not customized and they're not momentary. That is, they don't work right, replacing a precision process with a bludgeon.

And nobody seems to know the problem is low stomach acid!

So you'll hear that you shouldn't eat protein. This is bad advice in any case, but here it's off-target to boot. Don't avoid protein, just make sure your body can handle it.

Self-testing:

Here are a couple of tests you can do on your own.

- First thing in the morning put a teaspoon or so of baking soda in water and chug it down. It should make you belch. If you don't belch in a couple minutes you probably have low stomach acid. No guarantee, but that's a reasonable test.

- When your heartburn is acting up, when you are really feeling in your throat and in your chest, put a teaspoon (more or less) of either fresh lemon juice or cider vinegar in a glass of water, chug it down. If you have low stomach acid it should help. If you have high stomach acid you're not going to like me when you do that because it'll make it worse. Sorry.

So what to do?

Digestion plays a big role in health, so we really need to do something.

You might want to sip lukewarm lemon water. Squeeze half a lemon or quarter of a lemon into a glass of water with meals and that should help. Don't ice it down.

The other thing everybody should do is pump up your vitamins and minerals big time.

Most of us don't understand vitamins and minerals. For instance, if you're buying vitamins and minerals at the drugstore, you don't understand them.

It's not a matter of taking whatever. Most of them won't hurt you but what's the sense of taking them if they're not going to help you?

You might try bromelain. This well-behaved enzyme leaves your body in control of what's going on. It comes from pineapple and helps break down protein. You take one just before each meal.

Moving to Health includes more of the story on hypochlorhydria, low stomach acid.

Low stomach acid is common. High stomach acid pretty rare, so don't take antacids unless you know for sure you're dealing with too much acid.

Hashimoto's, Vitiligo and The Gang

"Bette, I have Hashimoto's and vitiligo, lots of sinus problems. Do antihistamines make auto immune diseases worse because histamine is a hormone? When I take them because of year round allergies my brain feels like it does when my thyroid levels are too low – are too high or too low. Can they affect your brain this way in a dizzy, spacy feeling? Thanks."

Unfortunately, your array of problems isn't unusual. That doesn't make it any less of a mess, but at least you know you're not alone.

Yes, antihistamines make things worse–because they beat up on your body. How so, you ask?

Well, your body creates histamine to safely handle allergens. Taking antihistamines, then, picks a fight with your body. Which is never a good idea.

Perhaps we should look elsewhere for answers. Both Hashimoto's and vitiligo can be related to low stomach acid. As can sinus problems.

http://BetteDowdell.com

You might consider it a clue that each of your problems is related to low stomach acid. A big clue.

Another thing to consider is that antihistamines lower stomach acid. If your Hashimoto's, vitiligo and sinus problems come from low stomach acid, you sure don't want to lower it even more.

And the brain-in-pain business? It's probably your long-suffering body begging for a little help.

Your body is way out of balance, and medicine doesn't do balance. That's up to you.

Setting up a solid vitamin/mineral program for yourself will take you a long way in the right direction.

We've been taught—mostly in advertisements and by doctors—that nutrition is weak stuff, but don't believe it.

A well-constructed vitamin/mineral program is powerful. And it doesn't just cover up symptoms as prescription drugs do; it moves you toward health

Getting your body parts all moving in the same direction will take effort, and I suggest you start with learning about vitamins and minerals.

Antidepressants and Other Bad Ideas

"Hi Bette This is a complicated question but here goes. I am hypothyroid. For awhile my antibodies were elevated. It looked like I had Hashimoto. After two years of exercise, healthier eating, less stress and supplements my antibodies went back to normal. I have had several doctors suggest that I have an adrenal problem as well, and that's very common. Vivian"

If you have thyroid problems, it would be uncommon not to have adrenal problems

"One doctor tested me and concluded I had orthostatic hypotension."

If you have adrenal problems one symptom can be that when you stand up your blood pressure drops. To test that, they take your blood pressure sitting and then you stand up and then they test it again.

If you get dizzy when you stand up, you probably have orthostatic hypotension.

"A holistic MD tested me and found out that at nighttime my excitatory hormones were high instead of low."

I don't know for sure what he/she means by that. Cortisol, an adrenal hormone, is excitatory, so perhaps that's it.

When the adrenals are perking right along, cortisol has a very specific pattern of release, including being low at night so you can sleep. If cortisol runs high at night, you have malfunctioning adrenals.

"Then I was put on a trial of low does Elavil for pain associated with peripheral neuropathy."

Now that is absolutely bogus. If you have peripheral neuropathy that means the nerves in your arms and legs tingle and burn, a very uncomfortable feeling. What does giving you an antidepressant do for that? Nothing.

It may be acceptable as an off-label use, but it doesn't do anything but cause damage. Doctors always want to put hypothyroid people on antidepressants.

http://BetteDowdell.com

Part of being hypothyroid is at least a little touch of depression, but the answer is to fix the thyroid, not shovel antidepressants down our gullets.

I remember some years back I was reaching for something. I should have had a ladder, but I was trying to stretch it out with a little milking stool—which scooted out from under me. I fell with a thud, with the joint between my leg and my hip catching the corner of the dryer.

I pulled more muscles than I knew I had. My doctor was out of town so I went to the doctor who was subbing for him and ended up with a "muscle relaxer."

Well, it turned out to be an antidepressant (which she assured me it wasn't). And it turned me into an instant banana.

Have you met people who are always stressed out because they just know terrible things are going to happen? That was me. All of a sudden. Take a pill, get maximum stress.

I took the antidepressant for three days. The last day, I was up all night, pacing the house making sure there were no fires and that nobody was dying in their sleep and that nobody was breaking in.

I mean I was gone, just totally over the top. It gave me a wonderful understanding of people who live with this kind of stress all the time because while I knew I was being illogical, I couldn't stop.

So as I was doing all my pacing, I wondered, as I wandered, what had happened to me, and I realized it was the medicine. So I stopped it, and the symptoms cleared up quickly.

"For three weeks I couldn't take any medicine, including my armour thyroid. It felt like I had about ten cups of coffee those three weeks and then as the Elavil went out of my system everything got better. I was tested for an adrenal tumor at the end of the three weeks and it was normal. High, but inconclusive. By the time I got the second round of tests the episode was over and the test was normal. Would the Elavil cause these problems?"

You bet your boots, and don't go back to that doctor. Elavil is murder on the endocrine system.

Antidepressants in general are really tough.

"By the way, the nerve pain I had disappeared when I discontinued a multiple vitamin with too much B6 in it. I spoke with my neurologist who said if you eat a lot of leafy greens and take a multi-vitamin too much B6 causes nerve damage and is sometimes irreversible."

Well, no.

First of all, our leafy greens nowadays don't have much nutrition in them unless you grow them yourself and you take pains to replenish your soil with minerals. If you buy them at the grocery store, they don't have much nutrition in them.

Multivitamins don't have too much B6 because they have the other Bs to balance the B6.

If you take a B complex, you have the synergy of all the Bs working for you, so you can handle more B6. Even a lot more. This is not common knowledge.

You mentioned the Carlson multi. While Carlson has lots of great products, that multivitamin isn't one of them. It's loaded with soy.

Soy is poison. For one thing it stomps on the thyroid gland. For another, it messes with the estrogen in men and women. No soy for you! Or anybody.

By the way, drinking diet soda with aspartame in it can cause peripheral neuropathy. So can eating anything with MSG in it or soy because they really pour glutamate down the hatch.

Aspartame and glutamate damage the part of the brain that controls the both the endocrine and nervous systems.

So your peripheral neuropathy could have come from diet soda. It's hard to say because so many things come into play, but you wouldn't be the first–or last–person to take that route.

http://BetteDowdell.com

What You Take Depends on Where You Are

"Dear Bette

I am always fatigued. I've been hypothyroid and had adrenal insufficiency since breast cancer treatment 20 years ago, and take Armour Thyroid and Cortef. Do you add other vitamins/minerals separately to your multivitamin or take the multivitamin only? I've been taking Natrol My Favorite Multiple Take One with Iron. I have consistently low ferritin levels and need to take iron. I am going to switch to the Twin Lab Daily One w/o iron. What iron supplement would you suggest if my ferritin continues to run low. I have also been taking separate B vitamins, Zinc, selenium, molybdenum, magnesium and fish oil. Am I overdoing it? Could the extra minerals plus the multivitamin be harmful? Thanks for your help."

A lot of people have thyroid problems, but few people understand vitamin/mineral supplements, so you're ahead of the game.

But consider a few tweaks.

The Natrol multi you take is average. I don't like the copper/zinc ratio. The calcium/magnesium ratio is too heavy in calcium. Especially since magnesium is far more important than calcium–despite all the calcium publicity. And the vitamin A is all synthetic beta-carotene, which isn't good.

I don't like a multi with greens in it. Too many people have trouble with greens and herbs. If you get a reaction, how do you figure out what caused it?

Your multi has boron, which is good.

Flavonoids are great, necessary antioxidants, but I prefer to take them separately so if I run into a sensitivity problem, I can tell which one did me in.

Taking iron is bad business, what with creating rust to gum up body parts, but at least this multi doesn't use a ferrous form. Eating beef (grass fed to avoid hormones and antibiotics) provides a great source of iron in the heme form, and your body won't over-absorb it.

The molybdenum you take does a lot of what iron does, but without the need to be so perfectly balanced. Molybdenum is amazing.

Since you've had cancer, you need to be sure you're getting enough vitamins/minerals of all sorts, but especially the mineral selenium and vitamin D3.

5000iu is a pretty standard adult dose of vitamin D3; if you haven't been taking any beyond what's in the multi, you might want to take a double dose for a few months, then get tested. You want to be at the high end of the normal range.

And since your cancer was breast cancer, avoid soy like the poison it is. Soy is terrible for the endocrine system, and breast cancer is an endocrine disease—with a strong soy link. (For you guys, the same goes for prostate cancer.)

Never take any B vitamin unless you also take a B complex. B vitamins need the synergy of the B complex, which avoids overdosing on any specific B.

Finally, no, you're not taking too many vitamins and minerals. Our bodies need all the nutritional help they can get, and it doesn't come from our food nowadays.

I don't know what brands of vitamins and minerals you're taking, except for the multi, and you may need some fine-tuning, but you're on the right track.

If your doctor adjusts your Armour to make the blood tests come out right, you're not getting enough, and that may be part of what's going on.

Undertreated hypothyroidism causes low ferritin (anemia). Fix the thyroid, and the anemia will take care of itself.

When doctors treated by symptoms instead of by the unreliable blood tests, patients took about twice as much Armour as doctors allow now—and they did a whole lot better.

The last time a doctor said my thyroid blood tests looked good, I was nearly bald and all but comatose on the floor. And I have to fight like a tiger for docs not to reduce my dose.

Unfortunately, blood tests rule—whether they make sense or not.

Bette's Story

A month before my first birthday, while driving down the highway to Grandpa and Grandma's house for Christmas, a drunk driver smashed into my parents' car.

Built in the days before seat belts were mandated, our little car had none.

My mother smashed through the windshield, then bounced back, her face hitting the dashboard—where she left her perfect teeth embedded. She suffered a traumatic brain injury, from which she never fully recovered—although doctors proclaimed her to be as fit as a fiddle.

My father hit the steering wheel with his ribs and the dashboard with his knees. While he couldn't walk for a while, he recovered.

Fortunately, my brothers (7 and 5 years old) and sister (not quite 3) were protected because they were playing on the floor in the back seat—which my father had suggested just moments before—to limit their energetic activities a bit.

I torpedoed, face-first, from my mother's lap into the car door. The impact tore the skin from my forehead, and I suffered a concussion.

Doctors didn't know (and still don't) that most concussions damage the pituitary gland, which controls the endocrine system, which, in turn, controls all of health. (Another thing doctors aren't taught.)

According to the docs, I was fine—within minutes after the crash, in fact.

But my mother realized something was wrong.

And so started my doctor visits, each of which ended with the verdict I was fine, followed by a little sermonette to my mother about not making a mountain out of a mole hill, as the saying goes.

But God bless my mother. She kept trying. (Note to doctors: Believe the mother.)

We moved a lot, so a new town meant new doctors, and maybe one of them would help. But, no.

Meanwhile, as the "She's fine" chorus continued, my health slipped away. By my early twenties, I was in very deep trouble.

For one thing, my brain became undependable. While teaching computer programming at IBM, I would suddenly forget–mid-sentence–why I was in the room. Given the army of people staring at me as I stood in the front alone, I was obviously teaching, but what?

I couldn't hold on to a thought. Speaking became a chore because I couldn't come up with the words I needed. Most of my hair fell out, and what was left changed color. I couldn't stay awake. I answered the phone in my sleep and never knew it.

My blood pressure was 70/40. My blood sugar was 46. My body temperature topped out at 95–on a good day. My pulse was about 50. I had Raynaud's Syndrome. Shingles arrived in force. And on, and on and on.

Doctors still said I was fine. One doctor suggested my problem was I wanted to get married. Another suggested my difficulties came from emotional problems he was sure all preachers' kids suffered. (I was too brain-dead to ask what problem all doctors' kids suffered.)

Finally, at long last, I found a doctor who took me seriously. One who had enough clout to do the right thing, whether or not it was the accepted answer, and recognized internationally for his diagnostic skills.

After several long office visits and more tests than I ever realized there were tests, he told me I had panhypopituitarism – meaning every part of my endocrine system was in a world of hurt. Big problem, no known cure.

But not long after I learned the news, we moved across the country, and I ended up back with "You're fine!" doctors. I realized it was up to me.

Okay, I can do this–especially with a diagnosis to give me a place to start.

And so I started.

But I sure didn't move quickly. It's hard to find information that contradicts what medicine wants you to know. The research may be fabulous, but if the conclusion offends the poobahs, under the carpet it goes.

It took me many years to figure out the entire puzzle. And I got hooked! In finding my healing, I discovered a calling to get excited about. I'm still digging around in the research, especially since the internet is setting free solid research that's been buried for fifty or more years.

I learned:

- How the endocrine system actually works, what makes it not work and what makes it work better. And, more importantly, that it controls our health.

- Our bodies falter without good nutrition–which turns out to be different from what we're told is good nutrition. So I studied a lot about nutrition–and found it improved my health much more than medicines.

  Nutrition includes much more than diet. Vitamins, minerals, amino acids and other supplements–whatever it takes to meet your body's needs–are essential. And they have to be quality supplements, not just any old thing you pick up at the grocery store, drugstore, Costco, etc.

- We're surrounded by enemies–toxins in the air and water, toxic artificial ingredients in our food, genetically-modified foods that do enormous harm to our DNA, and more. So I studied a lot about toxins. We can't get rid of all toxins, but we can lighten the load, which gives good nutrition the help it needs to win the battle.

So that's the stuff I write about.

Along with the 500-pound gorilla nobody talks about: Getting diagnosed. Diagnosis is a lost art.

Nowadays, doctors are required to diagnose via simple blood tests–many of which are unreliable.

The doctor who diagnosed my pituitary problem used tests–some simple, some very advanced–not to diagnose, but to support his analysis of my symptoms. That doesn't happen any more.

I couldn't get diagnosed nowadays because insurance companies limit the time a doctor can spend with a patient and which tests doctors can order. As you might guess, it's a money thing.

But without a diagnosis, how can we know what to do?

It's about symptoms–as it always has been. But nowadays we have to figure out what they mean for ourselves. So I talk a lot about symptoms.

Symptoms tell the story of your health. They are your body's way of telling you what's going on. And who knows your symptoms better than you?

The really good news is that our bodies want to heal. They fight like tigers to heal. Our role is to give our bodies the support they need to win the fight.

Resources

Too Pooped to Participate is a free, weekly e-newsletter containing health information you probably won't read any place else.

http://TooPoopedToParticipate.com

Moving to Health is a year-long, online coaching program that gives you the information you need to get and stay healthy. A whole new approach to health, it explains how your body works, what makes it not work, and what to do about it. Everything connects with everything in our bodies, and *Moving to Health* explains the connections. And it explains what our symptoms are telling us, which can be very different from what we've been told. And once you've figured out what your deal is, it offers direct links to quality supplements that can help—vitamins, minerals, amino acids, herbs and other supplements. (I receive no money or other benefit for these links. It's about you.) Good health means we need to understand what we're dealing with. *Moving To Health* explains it all.

http://MovingToHealth.com

Check out my Amazon author page to read about more of my books.

http://www.Amazon.com/author/bettedowdell

Understanding Blood Tests is a downloadable book that describes eight common blood tests and explains the results. Everybody needs four of the tests, while the other four are more situational.

http://UnderstandingBloodTests.com

Pep for the Pooped: Discovering the vitamins and minerals your body is starving for talks about what 31 vitamins and minerals do, how to spot deficiencies, etc. And it has links to quality products so you don't have to wander around health food stores asking questions. I receive no payment of any sort for these links; they're all about helping you. (This downloadable book is also a part of the *Moving to Health* program)

http://PepForThePooped.com

BetteDowdell.com is the place to go for links to everything I do.

http://BetteDowdell.com

Index

www.ingramcontent.com/pod-product-compliance
Lightning Source LLC
Chambersburg PA
CBHW050550280326
41933CB00011B/1794